Revolutionary Glucose:

Blood Sugar Balance Has the Power to Change Your Life

By:

Dr. Andrew S. Jones

Table of Content

Introduction

The Greek word for "sweet" is glucose. This specific type of sugar, which your body gets from the food you eat, serves as fuel. When blood sugar or blood glucose travels via your bloodstream to your cells, it is referred to as blood sugar or blood glucose.

Insulin is a hormone that moves glucose from the blood into cells where it can be stored and used as fuel. Blood glucose levels are higher in diabetics than in healthy people. Either they don't have enough insulin to get it through or their cells don't respond to insulin as they should.

Your eyes, kidneys, and other organs might become damaged over time by having high blood glucose levels.

The body uses glucose as its primary energy source. You obtain it primarily from the carbs you consume, such as sugar and wheat. Your body's cells take it up through the blood and use it as fuel.

Blood sugar or blood glucose refers to the quantity of glucose in your blood. Insulin, a hormone that transports glucose from the bloodstream and into cells where it may be used as fuel, helps your body control blood sugar levels.

If this procedure is disturbed, issues could arise. For instance, with diabetes, your body either produces insufficient insulin or fails to use it properly, which results in hyperglycemia, or high blood sugar. Hypoglycemia, or low blood sugar, can also happen. Serious health issues can result from both high and low blood sugar levels.

Blood sugar, often known as glucose, is the main sugar found in your blood. It comes from the food you eat and is used as your body's main energy source. Your blood supplies glucose to all of the cells in your body, which then use it as fuel.

Diabetes is a disorder when your blood sugar levels are too high. Over time, having excessive blood glucose levels may have negative effects. Even if you don't have diabetes, you could occasionally struggle with complications related to too low or too high blood sugar. Keeping a regular schedule for your diet, exercise, and medicine can help.

It is crucial to maintain blood sugar levels within your goal range if you have diabetes.

You might need to monitor your blood sugar several times each day. Your healthcare provider will also run a blood test called an A1C. It measures your three-month average blood sugar level. If your blood sugar is excessively high, you may need to take medicine or follow a certain diet.

This book describes what influences blood glucose levels and how the body produces and uses glucose. Additionally, it discusses normal blood sugar levels and the dangers of having high or low blood sugar.

Part I: what is glucose?

Chapter 1
The Significance Of Glucose
What is glucose?

When your blood sugar levels are under control, they frequently go unnoticed. However, they can have an impact on how your body functions on a daily basis when they grow or dip excessively.

So what exactly is glucose?

It is a monosaccharide, which is a form of carbohydrate that is the most basic and means "one sugar."

Other monosaccharides include fructose, ribose, and galactose. The body gradually transforms food glucose and other carbohydrates into blood glucose in this form.

Among the body's main fuel sources, along with fat and protein, is glucose. Both complicated and simple carb sources can provide people with glucose.

Depending on how quickly the body breaks down the sugar, carbohydrates are classified as simple or complex.

Complex carbohydrates provide a more consistent source of energy since the body digests them more slowly, according to the American Heart AssociationTrusted Source. They are therefore the healthier choice.

Uncontrolled glucose levels can have serious, long-lasting repercussions.

What is blood glucose?
Glucose, a type of sugar, is used by the body to create energy. This can apply to major structures like your muscles all the way down to red blood cells' molecular level.

In addition to the carbs we eat, our bodies also store glucose in the form of glycogen, which is found in our muscles and liver. Gluconeogenesis, a process that produces from fat, protein, and lactate, is another method.

In order for glucose and glycogen to enter our bodily tissues and be used as fuel, our bloodstream is essential. As glucose travels through our blood and circulatory system and reaches the required tissues, it starts to disintegrate. This is why the quantity of glucose that is in the blood is referred to as blood glucose.

Controlling the Level of Blood Glucose

While ensuring that our blood sugar levels don't fall too low (hypoglycemia) or rise too high (hyperglycemia) is essential to maintaining our health, delivering energy to our tissues and cells is equally crucial.

Our energy levels are maintained, we cease desiring sugar, and the chance of serious health issues including blindness, and heart attacks, and comes is decreased when our blood sugar levels are consistent and spikes are avoided.

Reduced insulin sensitivity, a hormone essential in lowering blood glucose levels, makes it more difficult for persons with type 2 diabetes to control their body's blood glucose levels. Due to this, persons who have type 2 diabetes need to take into account the variables affecting glucose levels since doing so will help to reduce the likelihood of any negative secondary health effects.

What causes variations in blood glucose levels?

Although a little amount of variation in your blood sugar levels is to be expected throughout the day, poor activity levels, dehydration, and stress can make this variation more pronounced.

Nutrition, particularly the ingestion of carbohydrates, is one of the main factors affecting glucose levels. Consuming excessive amounts of foods high in carbohydrates can significantly raise blood glucose levels since carbohydrates directly affect glucose levels. Although other macronutrients may also have an impact on your blood sugar, carbs continue to have the most power.

The Importance of Glucose

The metabolic processes that support life require energy, which is needed by every cell in the human body. A little, simple sugar called glucose is the main source of fuel for the body's energy production, particularly for the muscles, brain, and various other organs and tissues. Additionally, bigger structural molecules found in the body like glycoproteins and glycolipids are constructed from glucose. The glucose levels in the body are tightly controlled. Levels that are abnormally high or low have dangerous, possibly fatal consequences.

Brain Fuel

Normally, the brain gets all of its energy almost solely from glucose. The brain needs a steady supply of glucose due to its high energy requirements and inability to retain it. The body has several defenses against hypoglycemia or a severe drop in blood sugar levels. But if there is such a dip, the brain can start to malfunction. Headache, dizziness, disorientation, lack of focus, anxiety, irritability, restlessness, slurred speech, and poor coordination are among the common brain-related hypoglycemia symptoms. Seizures and coma are possible outcomes of a quick, dramatic drop in blood glucose.

Muscle Fuel

Depending on sex, age, and level of fitness, the skeletal muscles typically make up between 30 and 40 percent of the total body weight. During the activity, the skeletal muscles need a lot of glucose. Skeletal muscles store blood sugar in the form of glycogen, which is readily broken down to provide glucose during physical activity, in contrast to the brain. During the activity, muscle tissue also often absorbs a significant amount of glucose from the bloodstream. Despite the fact that skeletal muscles can use molecules generated from fat as an energy source, the depletion of glucose reserves during prolonged activity can cause rapid exhaustion, also known as bonking or hitting the wall.

Other Tissues and Organs' Fuel

The body's numerous organs and tissues have the ability to use a variety of fuels. Some other significant organs and tissues, in addition to the brain and skeletal muscles, depend on glucose as their main or only fuel source. Examples include the red and white blood cells as well as the cornea, lens, and retina of the eyes. It's interesting to note that although the small intestine's cells are in charge of absorbing glucose from food and transferring it to the bloodstream, they mostly use glutamine as a fuel source. This frees up more glucose for other tissues and organs that depend on the sugar more.

Structural Roles

The human body uses glucose, along with other chemicals, to create other crucial structural components in addition to its function in energy production. One such instance is the glycoprotein collagen, which has a protein backbone as well as simple carbohydrates like glucose. Skin, muscles, bones, and other human tissues all contain collagen, an important structural component. The growth and upkeep of the body's nerves are significantly influenced by other glycoproteins. Glycolipids, which are made up of the building blocks of fat and sugar, are essential parts of the membranes that envelop and support each of the body's cells.

Diabetic Hyperglycemia and Hypoglycemia

Because of the brain's exquisite dependency on a steady supply of glucose, symptoms of hypoglycemia often appear rather rapidly after a considerable drop in blood sugar. Hyperglycemia, or a high blood sugar level, may or may not have overt symptoms. The combination of high blood sugar and lack of insulin frequently results in signs and symptoms, such as — excessive thirst and hunger — unintentional weight loss — lack of energy — increased urination. Type 1 diabetics, who produce little to no insulin, frequently experience these signs and symptoms.

These signs and symptoms frequently do not appear or are not noticeable in patients with type 2 diabetes or its precursor prediabetes. Due to this, many persons with these diseases can go years without receiving a diagnosis. However, despite the absence of symptoms, continuous hyperglycemia can result in serious side effects, including kidney and heart problems, nerve damage, and eye issues that could result in blindness.

Precautions and Warnings

Discuss any worries you may have about your blood glucose levels with your doctor because glucose performs so many crucial bodily tasks. If you have any of the following risk factors for prediabetes and type 2 diabetes: — older than 40 years old — overweight or obese — sedentary lifestyle — parents or siblings who have diabetes

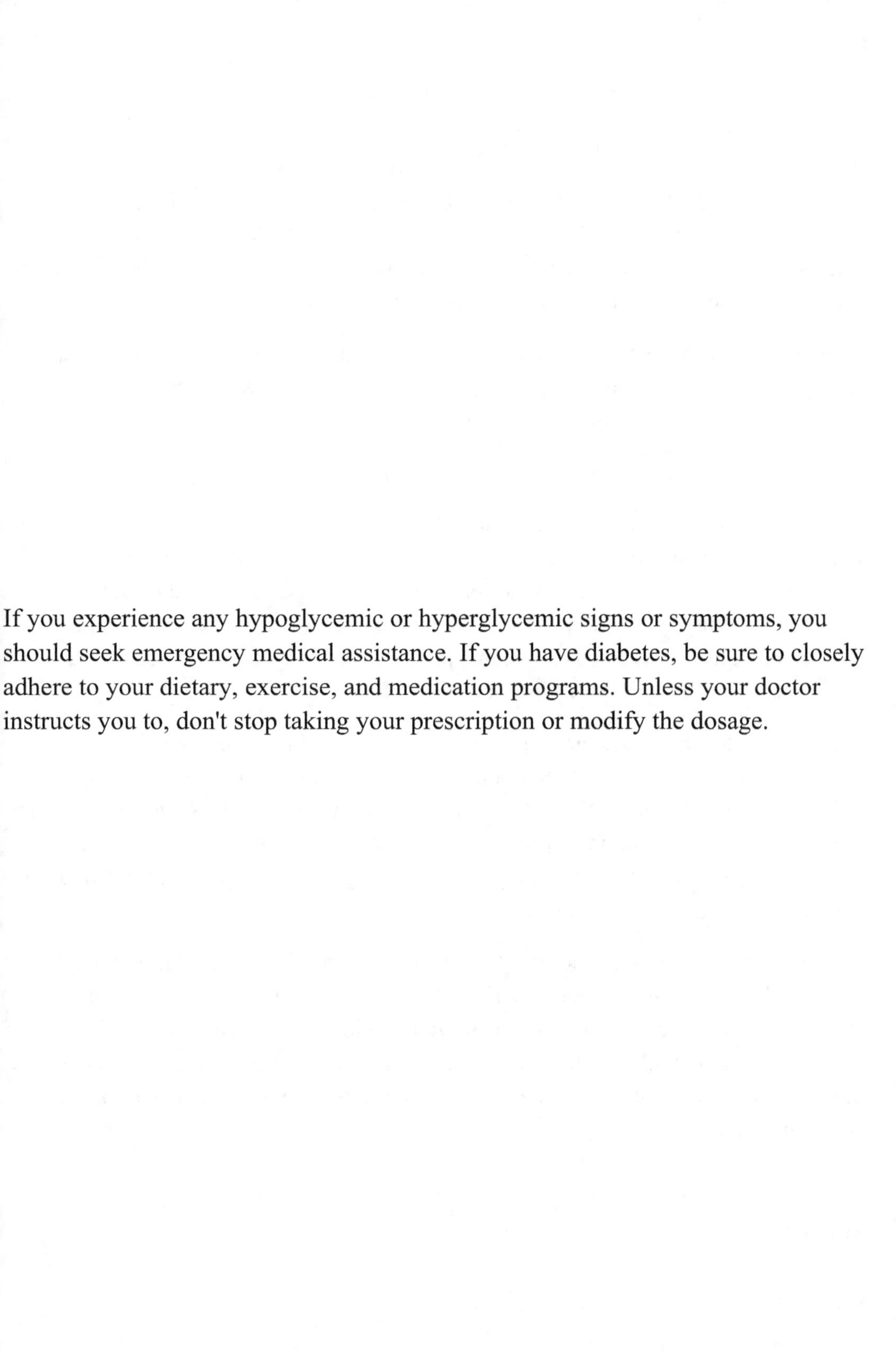

If you experience any hypoglycemic or hyperglycemic signs or symptoms, you should seek emergency medical assistance. If you have diabetes, be sure to closely adhere to your dietary, exercise, and medication programs. Unless your doctor instructs you to, don't stop taking your prescription or modify the dosage.

Chapter 2

How a plant produces glucose

The main sugar found in the blood and the main source of energy for people is glucose. The majority of it originates from carbohydrates found in foods like bread, fruit, and potatoes. The meal is broken down and released as glucose by the body's enzymes and acids after it has been consumed. After entering the intestines, it enters the bloodstream. Insulin then facilitates the entry of glucose into the cells.

How is glucose made and where does it come from? Glucose is created by plants during the photosynthesis process. A plant needs access to water, energy from the sun, and a source of carbon dioxide for this to happen.

Plants and Photosynthesis

Through the process of photosynthesis, plants produce food. It all begins when they use their leaves to capture light energy and take in water and carbon dioxide from the soil and atmosphere. Water oxidizes, carbon dioxide is reduced, and it obtains electrons inside plant cells. Water and carbon dioxide are converted into oxygen and glucose respectively in this process. While glucose molecules retain the energy, oxygen is released into the atmosphere.

Plants need this energy to grow, prosper, and produce other materials like starch and cellulose. Starch is stored in plant parts and seeds as a food source, while cellulose is used by these plants to create their cell walls. There is a lot of starch in some foods, such as grains and rice. Simply said, photosynthesis is a complex set of chemical reactions that uses oxygen from sunlight, carbon dioxide, and water to produce glucose, a simple sugar.

However, not all types of photosynthesis are the same. The most common one is C3, which creates 3-phosphoglyceric acid, a three-carbon molecule that eventually transforms into glucose. The resources available in a plant's environment determine the type of photosynthesis that develops. For instance, C4 photosynthesis increases carbon production while enabling plants to flourish in environments with limited water and light.

What Is Chlorophyll?

Chlorophyll, a uniquely colored pigment or colored chemical that the plant requires for photosynthesis, is present in the majority of plants in the globe. Actually, this chlorophyll takes solar energy and transforms it into chemical energy. The leaves appear green because it reflects green light while absorbing blue and red light from the sun. Plants stop producing chlorophyll, which results in the fall-like coloration of the leaves.

A plant's tiny chloroplasts, which are found inside plant cells, contain chlorophyll. Plant-based foods like broccoli and green zucchini, are both high in this vitamin. Foods that are more chlorophyll-rich tend to be greener. All plants contain one or both of the two forms of chlorophyll, named chlorophyll a and chlorophyll b. The two separate kinds of chlorophyll are both fat-soluble substances with antioxidant capabilities.

Contrasting Light-Dependent and Light-Independent Reactions

The two main stages of photosynthesis are light-dependent reactions and light-independent reactions, despite the fact that there are many other steps. As suggested by its name, the light-dependent reaction takes place inside the thylakoid membrane and requires a steady stream of sunlight. The light waves' energy is captured by the chlorophyll and transformed into chemical energy in the form of the molecules ATP and NADPH. The Calvin Cycle's light-independent stage, which takes place in the stroma, or region between the chloroplast and thylakoid membranes, do not require light, hence the name light-independent reaction. In this phase, carbon dioxide is converted into carbohydrates like glucose using energy from the ATP and NADPH molecules.

C3 and C4 photosynthesis

However, not all types of photosynthesis are made equal. C3 photosynthesis and C4 photosynthesis are two of the various forms of photosynthesis. The majority of plants engage in C3 photosynthesis. It involves the Calvin Cycle creating the three-carbon molecule 3-phosphoglyceric acid, which later turns into glucose. Contrarily, C4 photosynthesis generates a four-carbon intermediate product that, during the Calvin Cycle, breaks into carbon dioxide and a three-carbon compound. C4 photosynthesis has the advantage of generating higher levels of carbon, which enables plants to flourish in conditions with little water or light.

Can the Body Produce Glucose?

The liver serves as storage for glucose, helping to maintain steady amounts of circulating blood sugar and other biological fuels. In accordance with what the body requires, it can also produce glucose. The two hormones known as glucagon and insulin play a major role in controlling the urge to store and release glucose.

When you eat, your body produces more insulin and less glucagon, which encourages the storage of glucose as glycogen in your liver until you need it. Glycogenosis is the process through which the liver converts glycogen into glucose. By gathering waste products from the breakdown of lipids, amino acids, and biological waste, it can also produce the necessary glucose and sugar.

Consequently, the body does produce glucose, but it does so gradually. Instead, the body gradually holds onto the earlier forms of glucose, converting them into the actual glucose product when more is required.

Chapter 3
How glucose is absorbed into the blood

Starches and simple sugars are both types of carbohydrates that contain the molecule glucose, generally known as blood sugar. Because it is the brain's main source of energy and a substantial source of energy for all body cells, glucose is a crucial biological chemical. Glucose is transported from the digestive tract to the body's cells with the assistance of the circulatory system.

Function

Giving cells energy is the biomolecule glucose's main purpose. The glucose in the blood is taken up by body cells, where it is chemically burned to produce energy molecules that are used to carry out cellular operations. Some cells, including those in the muscles and liver, store glucose and release it when you're fasting. The most common carbohydrate molecule, according to Drs. Mary Campbell and Shawn Farrell's book "Biochemistry," is about glucose.

Transportation Issues

Several cell membranes must be crossed for glucose to go from the digestive system, where it is found after a meal, into the body cells, where it is used. Since cell membranes are composed of fatty substances and glucose is water soluble, glucose cannot independently cross cell membranes. Instead, transporter molecules must carry it into and out of cells. However, glucose does dissolve quickly in circulation.

Absorption

After being absorbed from the intestine, glucose initially enters the bloodstream. Drs. Campbell and Farrell explain that specialized cellular transporters known as sodium-dependent hexose transporters move glucose between the digestive tract's lining cells. Once glucose has passed through the intestinal lining, it is free to dissolve in blood and circulate throughout the body. After consuming a meal high in carbohydrates, blood glucose rises swiftly as a result of the intestinal transporters' speedy action. The blood glucose that was absorbed by the intestines is subsequently distributed to every region of the body by the heart's pumping function.

Cellular Ingestion

All body cells can be reached by glucose in the bloodstream, but it cannot enter them since accessing cells involves crossing a cell membrane, which glucose cannot do on its own. Two proteins aid in the entry of circulatory glucose into cells. The first is a glucose transporter protein or GLUT protein. The pancreas releases the hormone insulin into the bloodstream to aid cells in absorbing glucose from the blood as the second factor.

Expert Opinion

Since cells require insulin to absorb glucose from the bloodstream and since cells require glucose to meet their energy requirements, if insulin is absent, cells may chemically "starve" even in the presence of abundant glucose. This is the basic foundation for Type 1 diabetes, often known as diabetes mellitus. Without insulin, cells are unable to access the glucose in the bloodstream, which can result in a variety of symptoms, including cellular damage and death.

How Does Sugar Increase Energy?

A nutritional sweetener known as table sugar, sometimes known as sucrose, is generated from a number of plants, including sugarcane and sugar beets. Because sucrose is so simply and quickly digested and assimilated by your body, nutritionists define it as a simple sugar. Glucose and fructose, two straightforward monosaccharides, make up the disaccharide that makes up the sucrose molecule. Elson Haas, M.D. claims that glucose is the main type of fuel that your cells need to generate energy.

Digestion

You must digest and absorb sugar before your body can convert it to energy. Sugar, which is practically omnipresent in the American diet, is broken down into its two monosaccharide components, sucrose, and sucrase, very fast after consumption. Through the lining of your intestine, glucose and fructose are both easily absorbed by your bloodstream. They then go through your bloodstream to your liver, where fructose is converted to glucose. As a result, sucrose is a plentiful source of glucose that your cells may all use as fuel.

Cellular Respiration

Your liver contributes to the control of blood glucose levels and continuously supplies the energy you require. When your cells need energy, they take glucose from your blood and split it into two molecules of pyruvate. These molecules then move into the mitochondria, or "furnaces," in your cells, where pyruvate is converted to acetyl-CoA. The citric acid cycle and the electron transport chain are the two metabolic processes used in the mitochondria to metabolize acetyl-CoA. Adenosine triphosphate, or ATP, the energy source for all metabolic processes, is produced as a result. This oxidative metabolism of one glucose molecule results in the production of 36 molecules of ATP.

Storage Facilities

If you consume more sugar than your body requires for immediate energy, glucose turns into glycogen and is then stored in your muscles and liver. Excess glucose first transforms into fatty acids and subsequently into triglycerides, which are then stored in your adipose tissue once these organs have reached their glycogen storage capacity. Your body can swiftly break down glycogen to make glucose if the amount of glucose in your meal is insufficient to meet your cells' energy requirements, as might occur during a fast or physical activity. Similar to how triglycerides degrade into fatty acids and acetyl-CoA, which subsequently enter your mitochondria for "burning," triglycerides do the same.

Considerations

Sugar is a quick source of energy for your cells due to its simple digestion and high glucose content. However, one element fueling the obesity pandemic in wealthy nations is excessive sugar consumption. The average American consumes more than 150 pounds of sugar each year, and the normal American diet has around 32 additional teaspoons of sugar each day, according to the U.S. Department of Agriculture. The recommended daily intake is ten tablespoons. In addition to providing a variety of other beneficial nutrients, complex carbs, such as whole grains, fruits, and vegetables, supply enough amounts of glucose for your body's energy requirements.

What Purposes Does Lactose Serve?

The naturally occurring sugar called lactose, which is found in milk and other dairy products, is far less sweet than table sugar. While lactose's chemical components can undoubtedly be burned for energy, lactose doesn't have any special uses in the body; other carbohydrates can be burned without suffering any negative effects.

Chemistry of Lactose

Since lactose is a disaccharide, it is composed of two smaller sugar molecules. Your cells obtain their energy from the sugar molecules galactose and glucose. Drs. Reginald Garrett and Charles Grisham explain how lactase is converted into glucose and galactose when consumed in their book "Biochemistry." These little sugars are subsequently absorbed into your bloodstream, where they are then taken up by cells for use as fuel.

Using Sugars as Fuel

In a process very similar to how you can burn wood in a fireplace to release energy, the cells chemically "burn" glucose and galactose to release energy. The cells convert glucose and galactose into carbon dioxide and water by using a range of enzymes, which are substances that support biological activities. This process produces a significant amount of ATP, a chemical energy molecule that the cells use to power a variety of functions, including movement.

Special significance

According to Drs. Mary Campbell and Shawn Farrell in their book "Biochemistry," glucose can be found in a variety of foods, table sugar contains it, and starch is made up entirely of long chains of glucose. Therefore, you don't require the glucose from lactose to meet your body's energy requirements. Galactose can also be converted by your cells into glucose, which they do before using it as fuel. Therefore, you don't specifically require galactose in lactose. Although lactose is an excellent source of energy, it is not necessary for good health.

Additional Components

You can create one of two energy-storage molecules using the glucose and galactose found in lactose in addition to burning them for quick energy. Both glucose and galactose can be used by your cells to generate glycogen, which is a type of carbohydrate stored used by the liver and muscles. This offers a source of energy during times of fasting. Galactose and glucose can both be converted into fat for the storage of energy.

What Distinguishes Blood Glucose from Urine Glucose?

A basic sugar called glucose can be found in many different foods as well as in your blood. It has several uses, but its primary use as an energy source is crucial. Your body has delicate processes that work to maintain a normal level of blood glucose. However, when you have diseases like diabetes, your blood glucose levels might rise and cause glucose to leak into your urine. Although the blood glucose level is normally normal during pregnancy, glucose can sometimes be seen in the urine.

Glucose Sources

A simple carbohydrate, glucose can be found in many foods. In fact, almost all foods that include carbs contain glucose. It is possible for glucose to exist alone or in combination with fructose to produce the two-sugar molecule sucrose, also referred to as table sugar. Fruits and vegetables are additional sources of glucose. Large glucose molecules known as starch can be found in grains, legumes, nuts, and seeds. Additional sources of glucose include high-fructose corn syrup, molasses, honey, maple syrup, and honey. Fish and other animal products do not contain glucose since they do not have carbohydrates.

Glucose Functions

The primary purpose of glucose is to fuel your cells. After it is digested in your small intestine, it enters your bloodstream and travels throughout your body, where it can infiltrate the cells of every significant organ. During processes known as glycolysis and the Krebs cycle, which take place inside your cells, glucose is broken down and mixed with oxygen to create ATP, the body's primary source of energy. Adenosine triphosphate, or ATP, is a molecule that your body uses to carry out processes like recycling old cells and constructing new proteins.

Blood Sugar

According to "Maxwell Quick Medical Reference," the typical range for blood glucose is between 70 and 115 mg/dL. Your pancreas secretes the hormone insulin, which transports glucose into your cells where it can be used as fuel, in order to maintain the amount of glucose you consume within this range. Diabetes affects the pancreas' ability to secrete insulin, either completely or in sufficient amounts to fulfill your body's needs. Due to this, blood glucose levels might increase to exceed 1000 mg/dL, or 10 times the upper limit of normal, in the blood. When this occurs, some of the blood's glucose makes its way into the urine.

Glucose in Urine

Glycosuria, often known as urine glucose, is typically brought on by poorly managed diabetes. Healthy people may keep their blood sugar levels within the usual range, which prevents an excess from showing up in the urine. However, there are certain exceptions. Renal glycosuria often referred to as non-diabetic glycosuria, is a benign disease in which blood glucose levels are normal but urine glucose levels are elevated. According to "Current Medical Diagnosis and Treatment, 2011," this disorder, which affects as many as 50% of pregnancies, especially in the third and fourth months, has no symptoms. After birth, glucose usually stops being present in the urine, therefore no therapy is required.

Chapter 4
Why do we consume more glucose than before?

Even if a sugar-filled sundae or cupcake with icing on top may be irresistible, we should all be aware by now that sugar isn't exactly healthy. In fact, if you want to live a long, healthy life, it might be one of the worst things you can eat.

According to a UC San Francisco study, smoking cigarettes and drinking sugary beverages like soda can both accelerate the biological aging of your body. The effects of sugar on your body are much more complicated than just resulting in a weight increase. In reality, when you consume a lot of sugar, practically every organ in your body experiences stress, which is detrimental to your health in the short- and long term in particular.

This is what actually occurs in your body when you consume a lot of sugar, from an early insulin surge to an increase in your risk of kidney failure in the future.

Sugar and cocaine both have the same effects on your brain.

Dopamine and serotonin, which make you feel happy, are released in abundance after eating sugar. Using drugs like cocaine also has this effect. And after the initial high, your body desires more, just like with drugs. Gina Sam, M.D., M.P.H., head of the Gastrointestinal Motility Center at The Mount Sinai Hospital, explains, "You then become hooked to that feeling, so every time you eat it, you want to eat more."

Your insulin level increases to control your blood sugar.

Once you eat glucose, your body releases insulin, a hormone from your pancreas. Insulin's job is to absorb excess glucose in the blood and keep blood sugar levels stable.

After a short while, you experience the well-known sugar crash.

Your blood sugar returns to normal when the insulin completes its task. Which suggests you just had a sugar surge followed by a sharp decline that left you exhausted. According to Kristen F. Gradney, R.D., Director of Nutrition and Metabolic Services at Our Lady of the Lake Regional Medical Center and representative for the Academy of Nutrition and Dietetics, "That's the feeling you experience after overindulging at the buffet and being forced to do nothing except lie on the couch.

In fact, consuming too much sugar can cause extreme fatigue.

Being constantly tired, hungry, or thirsty are all symptoms of having consumed an excessive amount of sugar. Gradney adds that the physiological reaction of your body is to release enough insulin to handle all the sugar, and that can have a lethargic impact. You will also experience hunger and fatigue if you simply consume simple sugars since you aren't consuming enough of the other nutrients necessary to maintain your energy, such as protein and fiber.

You can start to feel like you're gaining weight.

The formula is quite straightforward: too much sugar plus too many calories equals too much fat. High-sugar foods not only contain a large number of calories in a tiny amount but also hardly any fiber or protein, which causes you to frequently consume a lot more than you realize you are. hazardous cycle According to Gradney, if all you're doing is consuming sweets, you can be gaining weight while also feeling ravenous. She continues, saying that consuming one candy bar and one 20-ounce soda every day (or an additional 500 calories) might easily result in weight gain of one pound over the course of a week.

Over time, consuming excessive amounts of sugar can cause obesity.

More than one-third of American people are clinically obese, and a large part of this is due to our high-sugar diets.

Additionally, obesity can cause insulin resistance, which raises blood sugar levels and eventually results in diabetes.

For unknown reasons, your cells may become less receptive to the effects of insulin when you're overweight or obese, making it more difficult for them to absorb blood glucose for energy. Your pancreas, therefore, produces extra insulin in an effort to compensate. However, even if the extra insulin is trying to do its job, the cells still do not react and absorb the glucose, which results in more sugar floating aimlessly in your circulation. Prediabetes is the term for blood sugar levels that are above normal. Blood sugar levels that rise much higher are type 2 diabetes.

By removing extra glucose from the bloodstream and storing it for later use, your liver plays a crucial part in the metabolism of carbohydrates.

Controlling blood sugar levels is one of the liver's roles. Your blood's glucose is used as fuel by your cells, and any extra is taken up by your liver and stored as glycogen. The liver will release glucose back into the bloodstream when your cells subsequently want energy, such as between meals.

However, your liver can only hold a certain quantity of glucose; the remainder can build up as fat.

Sam adds that if you consume more than this quantity, it converts to fatty acids and causes liver fat accumulation. When your body has more fat than it can process, it might develop non-alcoholic fatty liver disease, which results in the accumulation of fat in the liver cells. (Sugar isn't the only culprit, but glycogen storage and any sugar-induced weight gain are significant contributors.) Gradney states that fatty liver can appear within five years. However, depending on your eating choices and genetic susceptibility to insulin resistance, it can arise even faster. Liver failure may eventually result if it continues to advance. That's not really worth it, your love of Coke, is it?

In addition to harming your arteries, having blood that is heavily saturated with sugar can also harm pretty much every other organ.

It is essentially like trying to pump sludge down a microscopic tiny pipe while trying to pump blood that is full of sugar through blood arteries. "The pipes will eventually wear out. What transpires with your vessels is that "Explained Gradney. Thus, any organ dependent on small blood arteries may be impacted, including the kidneys, brain, eyes, and heart. High blood pressure and an elevated risk of stroke can result from it, as well as chronic renal disease or kidney failure.

Additionally, it damages your skin by destroying collagen and hastens the aging process.

Along with applying expensive anti-aging serums and SPF, reducing sugar intake can keep the skin looking young. According to dermatologist Debra Jaliman, M.D., "a lot of sugar in the bloodstream is affected by the collagen and elastin fibers in the skin." The body's proteins bind to glucose through a process known as glycation. This contains the connective tissue proteins collagen and elastin, which are in charge of maintaining the skin's smoothness and elasticity. According to studies, glycation makes it more difficult for these proteins to repair themselves, which leads to wrinkles and other aging symptoms.

Eating a lot of sugar causes tooth decay, as your dentist has likely already informed you.

According to Jessica Emery, D.M.D., owner of Chicago's Sugar Fix Dental Loft, "the sugar itself doesn't do any damage, but it sets off a series of events that can." "Our mouths contain microorganisms that consume the sugars we eat, and when this happens, the resulting acids can erode tooth enamel. When the tooth enamel is compromised, dental decay is more likely to occur."

Simply checking nutrition labels is a fantastic place to start if you're ready to cut back on your sugar intake. There is no "correct" amount of sugar you should be consuming, though, and that is a basic fact.

There are so many items that contain added sugar that you hardly even consider it (case and point: ketchup). According to Gradney, "We encourage consumers to read labels and check grams of sugar." The Academy does not have a strict recommendation for daily intake, she continues. A solid rule of thumb is to always choose the option with the fewest sugars. Choose water over juice or soda if you must." The sugar concentration is less concentrated in whole fruits than in juice, and the fiber makes it easier for your body to process. And to naturally reduce the quantity of sugar in your meals, choose whole foods. "The more processed meals you avoid, the better off you'll be."

Chapter 5

Discovering glucose spikes

When glucose, a simple sugar, accumulates in the blood, blood sugar levels spike. This occurs in diabetics as a result of the body's improper utilization of glucose.

High blood sugar: What is it?

The majority of the food you eat is converted to glucose. Because glucose is the main fuel for your muscles, organs, and brain to function properly, your body requires it. However, glucose must first enter your cells in order to be used as fuel.

Your pancreas secretes the hormone insulin, which allows glucose to enter cells by unlocking them. If you don't have insulin, the glucose just floats around in your bloodstream. Over time, it may become more and more focused.

Your blood glucose (blood sugar) levels increase when glucose builds up in your bloodstream. Organs, nerves, and blood arteries may become damaged over time as a result of this.

Diabetes patients have blood sugar rises because their systems are unable to utilize insulin properly.

High blood sugar signs and symptoms

Developing an awareness of the signs of hyperglycemia (high blood sugar) will aid in the effective management of your diabetes.

Some diabetics experience signs of elevated blood sugar right away. Others don't because their signs are nonspecific or moderate.

When your blood sugar rises above 250 mg/dL (mg/dL), you usually start experiencing the symptoms of hyperglycemia. As time goes by without treatment, symptoms may increase.

A blood sugar surge may cause symptoms such as frequent urination, weariness, increased thirst, impaired vision, headaches, and frequent urination.

A blood sugar spike: what is it?

When glucose accumulates in the blood and your blood sugar levels rise, a blood sugar spike occurs. This could occur after eating.

It's critical to understand the early signs of hyperglycemia or high blood sugar. Early diagnosis and treatment might lessen the severity of symptoms.

Early warning indications of high blood sugar can include thirst, a dry mouth, frequent urination, and blurred vision.

Ketosis and Ketoacidosis

If high blood sugar levels are left untreated for an extended period of time, glucose will accumulate in the blood and deplete your cells of energy. Instead, your cells will burn fat for energy.

Ketones are a byproduct created when your cells use fat as fuel instead of glucose:

• Diabetes patients are susceptible to diabetic ketoacidosis (DKA), an extremely dangerous illness when the blood becomes overly acidic. Ketone levels aren't kept in check and can quickly climb to deadly levels in diabetics due to poorly functioning insulin. DKA can cause death or a diabetic coma.

• Certain blood ketone levels can be tolerated by people without diabetes. The ketosis state is this one. Due to the fact that their bodies can still effectively use glucose and insulin, they do not go on to develop ketoacidosis. The body's ketone levels are maintained by insulin when it is functioning normally.

DKA symptoms and signs

DKA is a medical emergency that needs to be treated right away. If you notice any of the following warning signs or symptoms, call 911 or get emergency medical help right away:

• Sweat or breath smelling like fruit

• dizziness and vomiting

• Extreme mouth drying

• difficulty breathing

- weakness

- discomfort in the abdomen

- confusion

- coma

Blood sugar spike causes

All throughout the day, blood sugar levels change. Your blood sugar will start to rise as soon as you consume something, particularly items heavy in carbohydrates like bread, potatoes, or pasta.

You should consult a doctor about bettering your diabetes control if your blood sugar is continuously high. When:

(a) you don't take enough insulin

(b) your insulin doesn't last as long as you believe it does

(c) you don't take your oral diabetic medicine

(d) you need to modify the amount of your medication

(e) you're using expired insulin

(f) You don't follow your nutritional plan.

(g) You're taking certain medications, such as steroids

(h) You're experiencing physical stress from an injury or surgery

(i) You're experiencing emotional stress from issues at work, home, or with money

If you typically maintain good blood sugar control but continue to experience inexplicable blood sugar increases, there may be an immediate or more recent cause.

Consider maintaining a log of everything you eat and drink. Then, as directed by your doctor, check your blood sugar levels.

Recording your blood sugar levels first thing in the morning, before eating, and then again two hours later is customary.

You and your doctor can figure out what's causing your blood sugar to rise with just a few days' worths of data.

The following are typical causes of blood sugar spikes:

• *Carbohydrates:* Glucose is produced relatively quickly from carbohydrates. If you use insulin, talk to your doctor about your insulin-to-carb ratio.

• *Fruits*: The American Diabetes Association (ADA) recommends fresh fruits as healthful options for diabetics, however, they do contain fructose, a kind of sugar that elevates blood sugar. Fresh fruit is preferable to juice, preserves, and jellies.

• *Fatty foods:* The "pizza effect" is a phenomenon that can be brought on by fatty foods. Using pizza as an example, the fat and protein will not have an immediate impact on your blood sugar levels, but the carbohydrates in the dough and sauce will.

• *Sugary coffee drinks, electrolyte drinks, juice, and soda*: Take note of the carbs in your drinks because they all have an impact on your blood sugar levels.

•*Alcohol:* Alcohol also instantly elevates blood sugar, especially when combined with juice or soda. Additionally, it may result in low blood sugar some hours later.

• *Lack of consistent exercise:* Exercise on a regular basis makes insulin more effective. Discuss changing your medication to meet your workout routine with your doctor.

• *Overtreating hypoglycemia:* Overtreatment occurs frequently. To prevent fluctuations in your blood glucose levels, discuss with your doctor what to do when your blood glucose level dips.

Adverse Impacts over Time

The most common cause of long-term diabetic problems is persistently high blood sugar levels. Before symptoms occur, diabetes problems may steadily worsen over several years.

Serious diabetic consequences like heart disease, blindness, neuropathy, and kidney failure are more likely to occur when blood sugar is consistently high.

Ketoacidosis could also occur as a result of untreated high blood sugar. A diabetic coma or death could result from this urgent condition.

Your primary organs and bodily systems may be impacted if blood sugar levels are high for an extended length of time.

The following diabetes-related issues might also arise:

Eye Issues

Diabetes increases a person's risk of acquiring a variety of eye conditions, such as

•cataracts and retinopathy.

• glaucoma

A cataract is a thickening and clouding of the eye's lens that can cause impaired vision and reduce the ability to see at night.

The abnormal growth of small blood vessels that results in diabetic retinopathy harms the retina's blood vessels and is thought to be connected to long-term, untreated high blood sugar levels. Although the signs may not be immediately apparent, they can eventually cause blindness.

Glaucoma risk is increased by diabetic retinopathy. In this condition, the pressure inside the eye builds up, reducing blood flow and harming the retina and optic nerve.

Kidney disease

A gradual kidney condition called diabetic nephropathy causes the kidneys, which are in charge of filtering the body's waste, to stop working. It takes place when high blood sugar levels harm the kidney's blood vessels.

Early kidney illness may not show any symptoms, but it might eventually lead to renal failure.

Nerve injury (diabetic neuropathy)

Diabetes can cause diabetic neuropathy, often known as nerve damage. It is brought on by persistently elevated blood sugar levels.

Typically, symptoms develop over decades and are present gradually.

the four primary categories are a dependable source of information on diabetic neuropathy:

• proximal neuropathy

•focal neuropathy

•autonomic neuropathy

•peripheral neuropathy

Illness of the Heart and Blood Vessels

High blood sugar levels over time might harm your heart's blood vessels and nerves. Diabetes also increases a person's risk of heart attack and stroke, two conditions that affect the cardiovascular system.

Blood arteries can become blocked by high blood sugar if it is not treated. Foot ulcers and infections may result from this. In extreme circumstances, a toe, foot, or lower leg may need to be amputated.

Chronic Gum Disease

Gum disease, commonly known as periodontal disease, is more likely to occur in diabetics.

An increase in mouth sugar due to high blood sugar levels might have an impact on overall oral health. Diabetes increases the likelihood that a person may develop more plaque, spit less, and have poorer gum circulation.

Part II: why glucose spikes are dangerous

Chapter 6

What transpires in our bodies when we spike

You checked your blood sugar frequently when you first learned you had diabetes. You gained a better understanding of how several factors, including diet, exercise, stress, and illness, could affect your blood sugar levels. You've largely figured it out by this point. And then, bang! Something causes a spike in blood sugar. When you try to control it with food, exercise, or insulin, it dips dramatically. You're on a roller coaster that diabetics avoid riding.

Here is a brief introduction to how blood sugar levels differ between those with and without diabetes.

When you consume sugar, it enters your bloodstream where the hormone insulin from your pancreas helps it enter your cells to create energy. Your liver produces and stores its own glucose as a backup to assist keep your blood sugar levels within a reasonable range.

When you don't have diabetes, your body often performs a decent job of controlling your blood sugar levels.

However, the National Institute of Diabetes and Digestive and Kidney Diseases (NIDDK) states that if you have type 1 diabetes, which commonly manifests in childhood or adolescence, your pancreas generates little or no insulin to assist glucose absorption into your body's cells. That can enable your blood sugar to go too high (hyperglycemia). According to the NIDDK, elevated blood sugar is a symptom of type 2 diabetes, which often develops in adulthood and is caused by either insufficient insulin production by the pancreas or improper insulin utilization by the body. Headaches, weariness, increased thirst, and frequent urination might occur when your blood sugar levels rise above 200 milligrams per deciliter.

On the other hand, issues with managing your diabetes might cause glucose levels to swing the other way and become excessively low (hypoglycemia). A blood sugar level of 70 milligrams per deciliter or less indicates this, which might result in symptoms including shaking, fatigue, anxiety, hunger, irritability, sweating, or an irregular heartbeat.

Depending on their treatment regimen, people with type 1 and type 2 diabetes may check their blood sugar numerous times per day at home. Although there are alternative testing options available, this is frequently done with a portable electronic glucose meter that checks sugar levels with a tiny drop of blood.

Hyperglycemia and hypoglycemia are most common in people with diabetes, but they can happen to anyone.

Even if you don't have diabetes, a spike or fall in your blood sugar can make you feel awful. Simply put, it's unlikely to truly be harmful to your health in the same way that it might be for someone with diabetes. Both hyperglycemia and hypoglycemia can be fatal if neglected.

Obviously, you want to prevent significant blood sugar spikes or decreases. However, some factors can have an impact on anyone's blood sugar levels, while others are more of a problem for those who have diabetes.

Let's start by talking about four factors that can have an impact on your blood sugar, regardless of whether you have diabetes.

1. Your most recent meal or snack contained a lot of sugar.

Consuming a lot of sugary foods or beverages at once can cause your blood sugar to jump. It may be confusing to you if you don't consume a lot of foods that are plainly high in sugar, like cookies and candies, but foods like white bread and rice also include carbs that your body can turn into glucose, which can affect your blood sugar levels.

Eating or drinking too much sugar-rich food or beverage all at once might cause symptoms of high blood sugar, such as fatigue and headaches. According to Fatima Cody Stanford, M.D., M.P.H., M.P.A., an obesity medicine specialist at Massachusetts General Hospital and instructor of medicine at Harvard Medical School, these symptoms can appear if you consume less sugary food or if you have diabetes. So, while someone without diabetes could feel bad after consuming an entire bag of cookies, someone with the illness might only need one or two.

Including protein and fat with your sugar helps reduce the likelihood that it will significantly distort your blood sugar levels. Both nutrients can reduce how quickly your body absorbs sugar. They can also make you feel full, lowering the likelihood that you'll eat too many sweets to satisfy your hunger.

In addition, I advise people with diabetes to stick to their treatment schedule, particularly if they are aware that they are consuming more sugar than normal. If you're having a lot of difficulties managing your blood sugar, speak to a medical practitioner. You should check your blood sugar as often as your doctor instructs you to. To quickly lower a high blood sugar level, they may also offer a supplement of short-acting insulin or make food or pharmacological advice.

2. It's been a while since you last had food.

If you spend too long without eating, your liver can only make a certain amount of glucose before your blood sugar decreases and you start to feel woozy, weak or get a headache. While the ideal amount of time between meals varies from person to person, I advise against going more than five hours between meals, even if you don't have diabetes. Some persons with more severe forms of diabetes may need to eat roughly every three hours to prevent hypoglycemia. Consult your doctor if you're unsure of how frequently you should eat in order to manage your diabetes.

If you haven't eaten in hours and are already experiencing low blood sugar symptoms, you should at the very least grab a snack right away. If you don't have diabetes, you have a little more leeway to graze on whatever is nearby, however you should steer clear of foods high in carbohydrates to prevent your blood sugar from swinging too far in either direction. If you have type 1 or type 2 diabetes, I advise consuming 15 to 20 grams of a fast-acting carbohydrate, such as a half cup of orange juice, followed by another snack once your blood sugar levels have stabilized. A person with diabetes would not want to choose a food that is high in fat and protein in this scenario because doing so would actually decrease their body's absorption of sugar

3. You overindulged in booze.

Some alcoholic beverages, such as beer and hard cider, are high in carbs and may produce a surge in blood sugar. Additionally, excessive drinking without eating prevents your liver from releasing glucose from storage into your bloodstream, which results in low blood sugar.

If you don't have diabetes, your body will typically be able to resolve this on its own. However, having a well-balanced meal can aid in returning your blood sugar levels to a normal range more quickly. If you have diabetes and have a blood sugar crash after drinking, you may require a quick-acting carbohydrate to raise your blood sugar levels, such as fruit juice. Here, prevention is truly key. While dealing with diabetic patients, "we usually advise them not to drink too much alcohol and to make sure to eat a modest snack if they're going to drink alcohol."

4. You are using steroids.

According to the U.S. National Library of Medicine, corticosteroids are medications that imitate the actions of hormones produced by your adrenal glands. They are frequently recommended for problems like rashes, asthma, and autoimmune diseases like lupus and multiple sclerosis. They are typically used to relieve inflammation. However, corticosteroids can also raise your blood sugar levels.

Even if you were previously able to manage your diabetes well, using corticosteroids can make it more challenging. Long-term use of corticosteroids can cause steroid-induced diabetes or steroid-induced hyperglycemia, which is when someone without a history of diabetes develops the condition as a result of the medication. The theory is that steroids impact glucose metabolism by disrupting vital mechanisms involved in insulin and blood sugar regulation.

Ask your doctor whether you may switch to a medicine that works well without this side effect if you're taking corticosteroids and notice that you have signs of high blood sugar, such as exhaustion, frequent urination, and increased thirst. After you stop using the medications, your blood sugar will typically return to normal. Your doctor can assist you in developing a treatment strategy for high blood sugar even if you are unable to stop taking the corticosteroids.

5. You did not prepare before plunging into a hard workout.

If you suddenly go all-out in the gym without a sufficient snack beforehand, your blood sugar may drop and cause hypoglycemia, leaving you weak and unsteady.

Although anyone can experience this if they exercise and don't eat, the NIDDK states that it's more of an issue for those with diabetes who are using insulin or other diabetic drugs.

The other potential problem is that you might start burning fat for energy instead of glucose if your body isn't producing enough insulin and your blood sugar levels rise too high. This may result in the buildup of bloodstream acids called ketones, which can produce signs and symptoms like weakness and exhaustion, excessive thirst, shortness of breath, frequent urination, fruity breath, confusion, and abdominal pain.

This may develop into a potentially fatal complication known as diabetic ketoacidosis if untreated. When exercising with blood sugar levels over 250 mg/dL, diabetic ketoacidosis might develop more quickly.

Doctors often advise diabetics to check their blood sugar at a few important intervals when taking insulin, working out for a long time, or doing an extreme workout they aren't used to. This may apply to the 30-minute intervals before, during, and after exercise. You should eat a snack of fast-acting carbs if your blood sugar falls below 100 milligrams per deciliter in order to raise it to a range between 100 and 250 milligrams per deciliter. Don't exercise until you've reduced it back down to that safe range and a ketone test demonstrates that you don't have ketones in your urine if it rises beyond 250 milligrams per deciliter (you can find these over the counter or see your doctor).

Here's another factor that influences blood sugar levels, although it really only applies to those who have diabetes.

6. You either ingested too much, not enough or the incorrect amount of insulin.

You probably already know that type 1 diabetes requires lifetime insulin therapy to control your blood sugar levels. Injections or a wearable pump that feeds your body with insulin through a catheter can be used to administer this. And if you have type 2 diabetes, insulin may not always be necessary, but it may be helpful if a healthy diet and regular exercise are insufficient to control your blood sugar levels.

In either case, taking too much or too little insulin or not sticking to your medication schedule might result in blood sugar levels that are either too high or too low.

Whether your blood sugar is too high or too low will determine the best course of action. You can take the actions listed above to handle it in either situation, such as drinking fruit juice to raise low blood sugar levels or taking an emergency insulin supplement to reduce them (or otherwise following recommended steps from your doctor).

Ten Shocking Factors That Can Raise Blood Sugar

The power of knowledge! Be on the lookout for these unexpected factors that can cause your blood sugar to soar:

1. Sunburn-Pain makes people stressed, and stressed people have higher blood sugar levels.

2. Artificial sweeteners—although the additional investigation is required, several studies have found they can increase blood sugar.

3. Coffee, even devoid of sugar. Caffeine can make some people's blood sugar extremely sensitive.

4. Losing sleep—even one night of insufficient sleep can affect how well your body uses insulin.

5. Forgoing breakfast-can cause blood sugar levels to rise after both lunch and dinner.

6. The time of day – the later it gets, the tougher it can be to control blood sugar.

7. Dawn phenomenon-Whether they have diabetes or not, people experience an increase in hormones in the early morning. Diabetes patients may have blood sugar spikes.

8. Dehydration-When your body lacks water, your blood sugar concentration increases.

9. Nasal spray—some of these contain substances that cause your liver to produce more blood sugar.

10. Gum disease raises blood sugar levels and is a consequence of diabetes.

Chapter 7

How does spike make us ill?

You can't seem to drink enough water, your head is pounding, you're weak and weary, and your brain is feeling a little foggy. Sounds like a really bad hangover, don't you think?

However, if you recently overindulged in ice cream, it's probably not the case; instead, you're likely experiencing a blood sugar increase.

Sleeping it off is unfortunately not an option in this situation. Blood sugar spikes can be frightening and hazardous, so you'll want to find the cause of the issue as soon as possible (and maybe try not to spike those levels again).

What caused the significant rise in your blood sugar?

Your blood sugar may increase if glucose builds up in your system. This occurs when your insulin is unable to handle the excessive sugar intake.

People with diabetes frequently suffer blood sugar spikes since they might also be the result of insulin production being out of balance in the first place.

In order to maintain your health, glucose and insulin work together. Almost every time you eat, the food is converted into glucose, which enters your cells and becomes the fuel your body needs to function.

Your cells are designed to receive glucose with the aid of insulin. But here's the thing: if you have diabetes, glucose cannot enter your cells because your body does not utilize insulin well and does not create enough insulin.

When that occurs, the glucose lingers in your system and increases to potentially harmful amounts.

The frightening issue is that blood sugar surges can cause substantial long-term damage in addition to merely being uncomfortable. Chronic high blood sugar can lead to heart disease, nerve damage, visual issues, and renal failure if left untreated.

Additionally, it might result in ketoacidosis, a significant side effect of diabetes that should not be mistaken with the current trend of ketosis.

Long-term disregard for elevated blood sugar causes your cells to start using fat for energy rather than glucose, which results in the production of ketones. This typically isn't a problem if you don't have diabetes. However, doing so causes your blood to become overly acidic, which can result in a diabetic coma or even death.

To put it another way, you shouldn't play around with this.

What symptoms should you anticipate?

A person with high blood sugar will never feel great. You'll feel exhausted and weak at best, and you might even wind up in the hospital.

The following are some warning signs to look out for:

• excessive urination;

• exhaustion;

• increased thirst and dry lips;

• hazy vision;

• headaches;

• trouble focusing; and

• irritability

Long-term symptoms might range from low energy to repeated infections of the gums, skin, and vagina to slow-healing wounds and cuts to impaired vision.

You might believe that eating a lot of sweets causes your blood sugar to increase. That would make sense and provide a straightforward explanation and simple solution. Unfortunately, there are more variables involved.

Your blood sugar varies throughout the day and rises following the consumption of particular foods, such as carb-rich foods like pasta and potatoes. When it's regularly high, you should start getting concerned.

This could occur for a number of causes, some of which are unrelated to food:

• You either didn't take enough insulin or missed a dose.

- You neglected to take your oral diabetes medicine.

- You're ill or infected, such as with the flu or a cold. (When you're ill, your body releases chemicals to ward off pathogens, but these hormones can also inhibit insulin from functioning properly, causing a surge.)

- You're anxious more than usual.

- You overindulged in carbohydrates.

- You haven't been working out.

- A sunburn resulted from spending too much time in the sun. (This might hurt, which results in physical stress.)

- You didn't change your insulin dosage the previous night despite skipping a meal. (In an effort to correct the situation, your liver is overcompensating and has released an excessive amount of glucose.)

- There is a dawn phenomenon at work. Early in the morning, there is an increase in hormones that may have an impact on insulin secretion. Anyone can experience it, whether or not they have diabetes.)

- Your blood sugar is more concentrated because you are dehydrated.

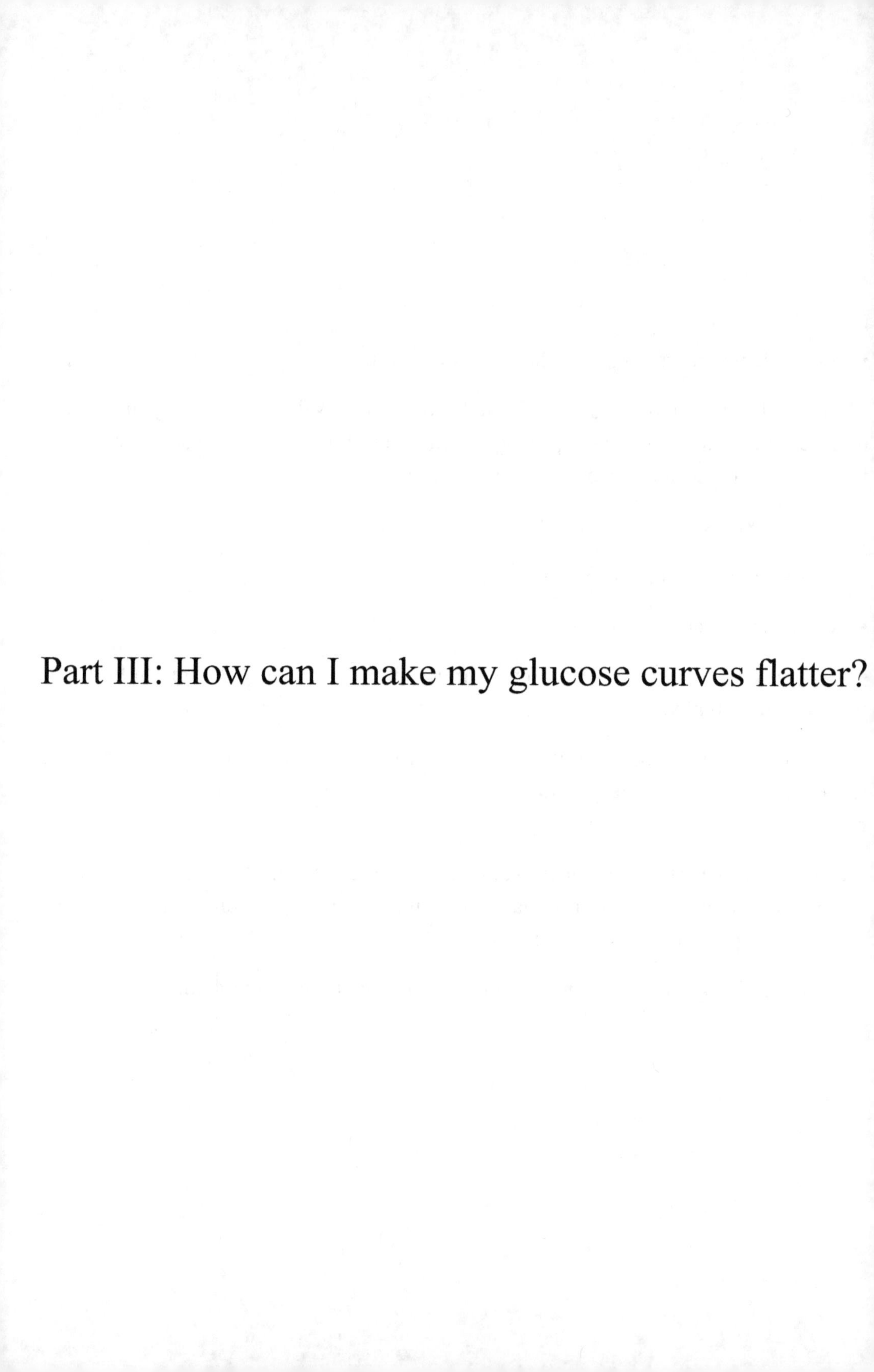

Part III: How can I make my glucose curves flatter?

Chapter 8

Eat your meals in the proper order.

Following a meal, a spike in blood glucose levels is completely typical. However, recent studies have discovered that the order in which food is consumed during a meal might affect how quickly the body releases glucose into the blood.

A key component of managing diabetes is controlling blood glucose levels, which is where nutrition and lifestyle decisions come into play. A normal mixed meal will include a variety of nutrients, such as proteins, fats, and carbohydrates.

The glycaemic index, which ranks foods based on how well they affect blood sugar levels, takes into account the kind and quantity of carbs in a meal.

The effect of consuming a meal's primary nutritional components first or last on the blood glucose response has been studied in a unique area of research.

The concept of eating the protein and non-starchy vegetable parts of a meal before the carbohydrates will result in a reduced glucose response is known as sequential nutrient intake. Consider serving the potatoes last and the steak and salad first.

An investigation of the effects of meal component eating order on blood glucose responses in 15 individuals with pre-diabetes was conducted by a research team in New York as an extension of the study into sequential nutrient ingestion.

The subjects consumed the same meal under carefully controlled laboratory circumstances three times, but the components of the meal were consumed in a different order each time.

One day, the protein and veggies were consumed 10 minutes after the carbohydrates. On another occasion, the carbohydrates were consumed 10 minutes after the protein and veggies. Vegetables came first on the third day, then protein and carbohydrates.

When comparing the glucose responses in the three hours following the meal, eating the carbohydrates last resulted in a lower and flatter glucose response than doing so first. Additionally, less insulin had to be secreted. This is beneficial for someone who is close to acquiring type 2 diabetes.

Why then does the glycemic response change when carbohydrates are consumed last? Though the exact mechanism is unknown, it is believed that eating fat and fiber first acts as a buffer to delay the breakdown of carbohydrates.

Implications

Eating a varied, balanced diet is crucial for anyone with diabetes or prediabetes, but this new study suggests that saving the majority of your meal's carbohydrates for last may have some benefits.

The ideal eating order is to maintain a healthy blood sugar level.

You may be wondering if eating a meal in a particular order truly makes a difference. Let the research speak for itself, then: According to scientific research, consuming a meal's components in a particular order can lower the meal's glucose surge by 75%. "So you're eating the same thing, but your body feels the effects considerably less," she said. Cool, no?

The following is the ideal sequence:

1. Vegetables come first

2. Proteins and lipids

3. Sugars and starches last

Do you want to know how this seems in action? Imagine that you are enjoying a home-cooked lunch with a portion of nutritious salmon, spinach, and brown rice, as well as a piece of cake for dessert (we highly suggest one of these Mediterranean-diet-inspired sweet treats). The spinach should be consumed first, followed by the salmon, the rice, and the dessert, in accordance with Inchauspe's philosophy.

However, Inchauspe suggests another blood sugar trick if you're dining out: avoid taking advantage of the free bread before a meal. She notes that those who consume the bread on an empty stomach cause a significant glucose surge. As a result, by the time they finish their main course, they are experiencing a severe glucose crash, are extremely hungry, and have cravings. That's not to say you should completely avoid the bread basket; if you wait to eat it with your protein, lipids, and vegetables, your glucose reaction will be much more stable.

Speaking of vegetables, try adding a high-quality greens powder with a good dose of fiber, like mbg's organic veggies+, to your home-cooked meals if you want to give them even more blood-sugar-balancing punch. This USDA-certified organic supplement contains a variety of rare organic berries, vegetables, and herbs, pre- and probiotics, vegan-friendly digestive enzymes, and hard-to-find sea vegetables like kelp and chlorella. This special mixture has the ability to improve digestion and support stable blood sugar levels. So eating your vegetables first can assist maintain blood sugar stability, but adding additional glucose-stabilizing effects from organic veggies+ on top can.

Remember that sugary beverages like sweetened tea might also have an impact on your blood sugar. Therefore, if you want to add a sweet beverage to your meal, make sure to save it as a treat and have it at the end rather than before (this includes natural sweeteners too).

Chapter 9
Halt the tracking of calories

Three things provide the calories in our food: carbs, protein, and fat. Carbohydrate calories can considerably affect blood sugar levels, in contrast to protein and fat calories. Concentrating on your daily carbohydrate intake might have a significant impact on your blood sugar levels. Knowing the right quantity of carbs that our body requires can be determined by checking your blood sugar two hours after a meal. Eliminating all carbohydrates is not the solution; rather, finding the proper balance depends on your calorie requirements. Finding the proper amount of carbohydrates for your body might be made easier by learning to count the carbohydrates you are consuming.

Starchy foods including grains, rice, cereal, pasta, corn, peas, potatoes, and soup beans are sources of carbohydrates. Additionally, all fruits and fruit juices, milk, yogurt, and sweets or desserts contain carbs. Blood sugar levels can be dramatically raised by juices, conventional soda, and other sweetened liquids. Understanding how much carbs are in portions of these foods requires reading the nutrition labels.

Examine your labeling.

The portion size mentioned on food labels should always be taken into consideration. Even though it might not be the quantity you really consume, this portion size is what all the numbers on the food label refer to. To find out how many grams are in the specified serving size, look at the total carbohydrate line item next. This is the weight in grams that will have an effect on your blood sugar. On food labels, sugars are also indicated, but they only represent a small fraction of carbohydrates. Any other carbohydrates that also affect blood sugar are included in the total carbohydrates, along with sugars. You may calculate the precise quantity of carbohydrates your body needs to maintain healthy blood sugar management by keeping note of the grams of carbohydrates you ingest in addition to monitoring your blood sugar levels.

The amount of energy in the food you eat is measured in calories. Whether or not losing weight is a priority for a person with diabetes, learning to calculate calories can still benefit their health. But according to a recent study, quitting counting calories aids in controlling blood sugar levels.

According to the International Diabetes Foundation, 537 million individuals (20-79 years) worldwide have diabetes. The number of people with diabetes will rise to 643 million by 2030 and 783 million by 2045. Adults with diabetes reside in nations with low and medium incomes.

Type 2 diabetes is clearly correlated with lifestyle factors such as inactivity, aging, obesity, and modernization. We currently face a significant global public health problem in the prevention of type 2 diabetes. According to experts, the "Diabesity" epidemic—which includes both obesity and type 2 diabetes—is likely to be the worst in recorded human history.

According to several clinical investigations, decreasing 5–10% of one's body weight aids with blood sugar regulation. Yes, your BMI is important, but merely adding or subtracting calories from your diet won't have any effect.

Calories In vs. Calories Out: What Are They?

This theory is predicated on the premise that when there is a calorie deficit, the body must make up the difference by burning stored fat. The idea is based on the idea that you will lose weight if you consume fewer calories than you burn. In plain English, "calories in" refers to the calories gained from the food eaten, while "calories out" refers to the number of calories expended during exercise.

To put it simply, the body uses the calories you eat to fuel your basal metabolic rate (BMR), digestion, and physical activity. According to Poojitha L. Acharya, if you consume the same number of calories as you expend each day, your weight will remain stable.

Instead of tracking calories, she advises concentrating on overall nutrition and wellness through the quality of food rather than being fixated on specific figures.

Make informed decisions on what to eat:

The number of calories in a slice of white bread and a slice of whole-grain bread are the same, but they are not the same. In comparison to white bread, whole-grain bread has four times as much potassium, three times as much zinc, and twice as much protein and fiber.

Blood sugar management and food intake are tightly related. Your blood sugar will increase if you eat more than is advised on your meal plan. Although diets high in carbohydrates (carbs) have the greatest effect on blood sugar levels, all foods' calories have an impact as well.

Pay attention to what you consume, especially the amount size. The amount of food you consume has a significant impact on how your body processes it and how it affects your blood sugar.

Important For Diabetes Care

1. Put quality of nutrition first rather than counting calories. Avoid processed foods, and increase your daily intake of fruits and vegetables. Consume fruits and vegetables as nature intended or prepare them using fat-free or low-fat methods. Choose fresh fruit over canned or juiced varieties.

2. Keep moving and exercise frequently. To stay physically active, strike a balance between exercises, walking, jogging, and yoga. The prevention and management of insulin resistance and prediabetes rely heavily on exercise. Aerobic and resistance training both improve insulin action, at least temporarily, and can help with the management of BG levels, lipids, blood pressure, CV risk, mortality, and QOL. However, exercise must be done regularly to reap the benefits, and this is likely to include regular training of various kinds.

3. Make sure you get enough sleep and stick to a strict routine. Weight gain may result from insufficient sleep or sleep rhythms that are not in line with the body's regular daily cycles. The body's numerous organs and organ systems will benefit from maintaining a circadian rhythm.

4. Seek professional advice for better direction. Gain knowledge from their exposure, experience, training, and practical experience. With their smartphone glucometers and qualified advice from doctors and coaches, a number of apps, like BeatO and others, have clinically proven programs to help control and reverse diabetes. Find out from friends which software or how-to manual worked best for them.

5. The best strategy to control blood glucose levels and prevent diabetes complications is to follow a healthy eating plan. Dietician Poojitha L. Acharya advises tailoring the diet to your unique needs if you need to lose weight (BeatO App, Diabetes Care Coach).

Chapter 10
Reduce the breakfast curve.

You are well aware of the significance of blood glucose and why preserving your general health depends on it. But if you're new, don't worry! A concise summary of everything you need to know is provided below.

Blood glucose levels in your body fluctuate naturally. As food is digested and taken into your bloodstream, they rise after each meal and falls as your cells absorb the glucose for cellular energy. We refer to this rising and falling pattern as the blood glucose curve.

However, not all curves are made equally. Numerous variables might cause glucose levels to rise and fall at quicker or slower rates. These variables include food, physical activity, genetics, microbiota, and more, and these variations can have a surprisingly significant effect on your general health.

Short-term side effects of these abrupt blood glucose rise include increased fatigue, irritability, and desire susceptibility. Long-term, this imbalance may result in weight gain, cardiovascular issues, and ultimately, more severe medical ailments.

It's not surprising that your food is one of the finest methods to focus on optimizing those curves since eating is the immediate catalyst for growing blood glucose levels.

Let's start hacking to flatten your glucose curve.

Let's get to those hacks you've been waiting for without further ado.

There are many healthy eating suggestions that can help your blood sugar, but we've selected the top 5 ideas so that anyone can use them. Some of them might even be things you already do, in which case congrats! It appears that you have already completed some homework.

Hack #1: Pick goods that are fiber-rich and unsweetened.

All plant-based foods, including grains, beans, and fruits, vegetables, are important sources of fiber. But unlike other components of your diet, your body doesn't truly digest it; instead, it goes through your system undigested. If you've never heard of fiber before, you might be unclear as to why you would need it. Actually, fiber has a major impact on how efficiently your digestive system functions. Since it isn't absorbed, it helps to smooth bowel motions and flush waste out of your gut, keeping you on a regular schedule.

Additionally, these dietary fibers offer carbohydrates shape, which slows down the breakdown and absorption of carbohydrates.

Simple added sugars, on the other hand, cause blood glucose levels to rise more quickly because they are absorbed into the bloodstream considerably more quickly.

For instance, make an effort to include more organic, high-fiber, and low-carb foods in your meals. You can top your yogurt with delectable seasonal berries and chia seeds or swap your regular white toast for a filling whole-grain option.

Hack #2: Combine your carbohydrates with proteins and a few fats.

It's dull and unhealthy to limit your meal to just one food category.

Due to their rapid digestion, carbohydrates have a significant role in how quickly our blood glucose levels start to rise. Increasing variety by including additional protein and a small amount of fat will lessen those glycemic reactions. [2] Because protein and fat take longer to digest than carbs, they raise blood sugar levels more gradually when included in a meal.

These various eating habits can also encourage the release of insulin, which is a crucial stage in your body's normal blood sugar regulation.

For instance, mix up your plate! Instead of loading up on a big bowl of pasta, add some vegetables and fish to your meal.

Hack #3: The order of your meals counts.

Start with vegetables and protein, then move on to carbs. Your post-meal glucose reaction can be significantly reduced by up to 73% if you eat your veggies and/or protein 15 minutes before you consume items high in carbohydrates. [3] Your body will appreciate that you prioritized those fiber-rich vegetables and slow-digesting proteins, as we discussed in the previous two hacks.

Example: For dinner, start with a simple salad and some chicken. Give yourself enough time to enjoy every bite. After you've had time to digest, switch to a food with more carbohydrates, like rice or pasta. Additionally, if your main meal includes a salad or veggies, start with those.

Hack #4: Include a little vinegar

When ingested with carbohydrates, vinegar has been demonstrated in recent research to improve blood glucose levels. Two spoonfuls a day is all it takes to make a difference.

Although the science is still in its infancy, it is thought that vinegar can enhance glucose uptake following a meal high in carbohydrates, hence assisting in blood sugar stabilization.

Say goodbye to store-bought dressing, for instance. Instead of dousing your healthful salad in a heavy layer of sweet, dairy-based dressing, add vinegar and a little light spice.

Hack #5: Consuming fermented foods can feed your microbiome

Probiotic-rich fermented foods encourage the growth of intestinal bacteria—the good kind, we guarantee! Kefir, a fermented milk beverage, was the subject of one particular study that discovered the drink can also support normal glucose levels. It has been demonstrated that the yogurt-like beverage lowers blood sugar and insulin baseline levels.

Kefir, for instance, can be a star ingredient if you don't like the sour flavor. Kefir is popular as a pleasant drink on its own. Add some kefir to your smoothie for a probiotic boost or use it as the creamy base for a vegetable dip.

In order to flatten the glucose curve, a balance must be reached.

It may take some practice to get the hang of paying attention to when what, and how you eat, especially if you're new to it.

It's OK to concentrate on one step at a time as you begin your trip, getting a sense of what works for you.

Feel free to include these suggestions in your daily routine as they are a fantastic place to start for a more mindful diet. Find a strategy that suits you. One of the many lifestyle choices that affect blood sugar levels is eating habits. You have the power to make eating decisions.

Chapter 11
Prior to eating, get some vinegar.

The ability of acidic beverages to boost glycemic control has recently received a lot of attention. Let me share with you what the science has to say about these beverages and their effects on our daily carbohydrate intake, though, before you grab the bottle of vinegar.

What is vinegar?

Aqueous vinegar is a versatile and tasty product of the anaerobic fermentation of carbohydrates by yeasts into ethanol and the subsequent aerobic bacterial oxidation of ethanol into acetic acid. Around 5000 B.C., this naturally fermented substance was discovered for the first time in Egyptian urns and Babylon. Since then, numerous cultures have utilized it as a condiment, food preservative, wound healer, and sour drink.

Vinegar can also be created from rice, wheat, and other fruit liquids like apple, grape, and coconut juice. The name vinegar is derived from the Old French vin aigre, which means sour wine. Over time, the food industry expanded the use of vinegar in a variety of acetic acid-related items, including salad dressings, pickled goods, and recipes using sourdough.

Starchy foods' negative effects on blood sugar are lessened by vinegar.

Starches are a class of complex carbohydrates made up of several linked simple sugars, such as bread, cereal, and pasta. When we consume starchy meals, our body converts them into glucose, which, once it reaches the circulation, is used for energy. In a healthy person, this causes brief insulin rises; however, persistent blood sugar spikes might result in lethargy and hunger. They might eventually cause metabolic diseases like type 2 diabetes.

According to several studies, taking vinegar either before or in addition to starchy foods like bread, rice, bagels, and cereal bars can assist both healthy adults and people with glucose problems avoid post-meal glucose increases.

For instance, consuming 20 grams of apple cider vinegar (about 1.5 US tbsp) in a glass of water before consuming a bagel with juice cut the amount of blood glucose rise that occurred during the meal in half. Consuming vinegar with white bread also helped to prevent blood sugar increases after meals. 20–35% less blood sugar was produced when rice was consumed with pickled foods or 11 grams of vinegar, or about 3/4 of a US tbsp. Blood sugar levels were lowered by 20% when 30 mL of vinegar, or 2 US tbsp, was diluted in water and consumed five minutes before a starchy meal. Consumption of lemon juice appears to lessen the glycemic response to bread.

How can vinegar lower blood sugar spikes?

The acidic qualities of vinegar are linked to its advantages in lowering blood sugar rises. The enzyme salivary-amylase, which is stable when the pH is between 4.5 and 7.0, begins the process of breaking down starch in the mouth. Once in the stomach, enzymatic digestion continues until salivary-amylase is inactivated by the stomach's growing acidity (pH between 3.0 and 3.8). Other enzymes that can successfully act in an acidic environment continue the digestion process. Following the completion of starch digestion, glucose is eventually absorbed and delivered into the bloodstream in the small intestine.

Up to half of the starch from bread can be digested by -amylase within the first 30 minutes of gastric digestion before the acidic environment of the stomach inactivates it. However, eating foods with vinegar or lemon at the same time speeds up the inactivation of -amylase, reducing the release of glucose until small intestine digestion is complete. In the end, this reduces the quantity of glucose that enters the bloodstream. Blood sugar levels are reduced by 20–50% when starchy meals are combined with vinegar, pickled items, or lemon juice.

Vinegar may reduce appetite and lengthen your feeling of fullness.

Studies with a single vinegar exposure demonstrated that drinking vinegar with meals reduced hunger in a mixed group regardless of age or health status for up to 2 hours after a meal. Another study discovered that vinegar increases sensations of fullness. It can take longer for food to leave the stomach when acidic drinks are consumed with starchy meals.

These findings are encouraging because they suggest that simply consuming starchy foods with vinegar or lemon beverages may help you avoid feeling hungry right away and may even boost your energy and happiness after eating.

Advice on how to make your meals sour

To reduce glucose spikes and optimize your glycemic profile, try adding about 1-2 teaspoons of vinegar as a dressing or diluted in beverages, or sipping a glass of lemon juice while eating. You can drink vinegar with meals as a salad dressing, together with a meal that contains starches, or diluted in a glass of plain water.

A dose per meal of roughly 10-30 grams, or 2-6 tablespoons, of apple cider, wine, and grape vinegar are other acidic supplements that have been employed in research.

Is it okay to eat vinegar?

It's important to stress that these tiny amounts of vinegar and lemon juice are safe for the digestive epithelium because their pH levels (both of which range from 2-3) are similar to those of gastric juice and a number of commercially available acidic drinks like Colas, Tonic waters, and sports drinks. On the other hand, taking too much can be dangerous and result in a number of serious adverse effects, such as stomach ulcers.

Conclusion

To survive, every cell in the human body needs glucose. However, the body can also suffer if it consumes too much glucose. The control of hormones is how the body keeps this balance. When blood glucose levels are high, the body will release insulin to let the sugar enter cells. Glucagon will be released if the blood glucose level is insufficient. The production of glucose and the release of glucose reserves are both triggered by this hormone. The sympathetic nervous system will activate if the body perceives a threat. The release of adrenaline, which triggers haptic glucose release, is a component of this reaction. If the body is unable to control blood glucose levels effectively, diabetes may be present. The primary cause of diabetes type 1 is an inability to make insulin. Insensitivity to insulin is the cause of diabetes type two. Alcohol, which also has a generalizing effect on the body, is bound to cause a reaction since blood glucose regulation systems to have a significant impact on the body. Blood glucose levels may initially raise, but only in the case of alcoholic beverages heavy in carbohydrates, such as beer. Alcohol metabolism causes glucose to be converted to pyruvate, which causes blood glucose levels to fall. A decrease in blood sugar is also likely a result of alcohol's impact on judgment.

Diabetes is a slowly fatal disease for which there are no recognized cures. However, with the right knowledge and prompt treatment, its problems can be minimized. Heart attack, kidney damage, and blindness are three serious side effects. For patients to avoid complications, it's critical to maintain careful control over their blood glucose levels. One of the challenges with strict blood glucose control is that such efforts may result in hypoglycemia, which causes considerably more serious problems than an elevated blood glucose level. The hunt for alternate diabetes treatment strategies is now underway. This book seeks to provide a broad overview of the state of diabetes research today. I hope to inspire future researchers to take on the problems since I see diabetes as one of the most difficult study areas of the twenty-first century.